Silent
Inheritance

Silent Inheritance

Are You Predisposed to Depression?

Susan Rex Ryan

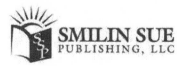

DISCLAIMER

Published in November 2017 by Smilin Sue Publishing, LLC.

smilinsuepubs.com

Publisher's Cataloging in Publication Data

ISBN: 9780984572021

Cover design by BookWise Designs.

Editing by Jessica of CreateSpace.

Printed in the United States of America.

ISBN: 0984572023

Dedication

With all my heart, to those who seek solutions to depression.

Contents

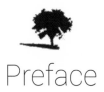

Preface

When I wrote my first book *Defend Your Life* about the health benefits of vitamin D3, my goal was to help people feel better and enjoy improved overall physical health by obtaining adequate vitamin D3. At that time, however, I did not focus my research and writing on mental health issues.

A few years later, I began to connect additional dots, not only between vitamin D3 and the brain, but how genetic predispositions may affect how we think and behave. My own experiences with depression inspired me to share them in this book.

Silent Inheritance guides you to find out and understand your genetic predispositions related to depression, and how to potentially overcome them by using nutritional and conventional means.

The first part of *Silent Inheritance* explains basic information about depression. The second part examines genetic predispositions for depression, including how to test for them. It also addresses neurotransmitters and genetic variants that can affect depression. The third part presents nutritional and conventional means to alleviate inherited depression.

Reading this book will to help you understand how your DNA and other external factors influence depression that you may have silently inherited from your biological parents. Moreover, you may gain a fresh perspective of why you behave the way you do and how to manage that behavior. Finally, you can learn how to fight the stigma that surrounds depression.

Life is too precious to ignore depression. Please remember: you are not alone. There is helpful information—right here!

Susan Rex Ryan

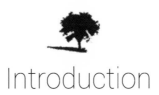

Introduction

n slightly less than a year, my emotional worlds collided. Depression reigned. But happiness ultimately won.

Decades of self-induced and environmental stress finally pushed my DNA over the edge—I was diagnosed with mild-to-moderate depression at the age of sixty-two.

Depression, for me, was terrifying. I felt that I had fallen deeply in an abyss of unrelenting horror. Despite being surrounded by love, I felt little comfort.

But, fortunately, I recognized that my thoughts and behavior were not really me.

They were apparitions of my mind, cultivated by imbalances in my brain.

My brain was telling me things of which I wanted no part. Thankfully, I came to understand that I had inherited this condition and resolved to overcome it.

I am convinced that inherent irregularities in our DNA render us vulnerable to depression. However, so does our environment, including the air we breathe, the food and water we consume, as well as the daily stresses of life, some of which we can control.

Chapter 1

Introduction to Depression

You do not know how much I hesitated to write this book. I knew that I needed to tell my story, but admitting to anyone on the planet that I have depression was, and still is, difficult.

The stigma of depression hangs over society like an endless collection of dark rain clouds. It is, however, acceptable to have an illness in almost any organ of our body except the brain. Having something "wrong" with our brains is something that can make us be shunned by most people.

Over 350 million people of all ages globally suffer from depression, according to the World Health Organization. Yet few truly understand this condition. Moreover, modern medicine is still grasping for effective treatments. The truths of depression remain hidden behind vaulted doors, awaiting the keys.

For decades—until I suffered from depression—I viewed it with haughty judgment that it was a sign of weakness. Depressed people were to be avoided or at least dealt with deliberately. Who needs to be around someone who is depressed?

My experience with depression firmly put me in my place. Oh, and did I learn firsthand about the absolute horrors of depression! Awful thoughts without thinking. Bad visions without seeing. Actions without feeling.

Count yourself fortunate if you have never been depressed. But please understand that hundreds of millions of the people have gene variants that could be switched on, bringing depression symptoms. Nonetheless, you can learn about your predisposition to depression and act accordingly to minimize the risk of turning on your "depression genes."

If you are, or have been, depressed or have depression in your family, consider finding out your genetic predisposition. *Silent Inheritance* guides you to understand what your gene variants are and the environmental factors that are most likely turn on depression. Then you can learn how to diminish your depression so that you can improve your quality of life.

First, let's look at symptoms that may be indicative of inherited depression.

Chapter 2

Major Depression Symptoms

I n this book I focus on probable genetic depression that is most likely triggered by the stress of epigenetics (see chapter 9). Please understand that genetic depression differs from usual mood fluctuations and temporary emotional responses to daily challenges.

The World Health Organization (WHO) describes depression as a *recurrent* disorder that involves repeated, if not chronic, depressive episodes over an extended period of time.

The positive news about depression is that it is among the most treatable of psychiatric diseases. Unfortunately, many people unknowingly suffer from depression and do not seek treatment. Untreated depression, in some cases, leads to suicide. According to multiple sources, more than 50 percent of people who die by suicide suffer from major depression.

The fifth edition of an imposing reference book called the *Diagnostic and Statistical Manual of Mental Disorders (DSM-V)* represents the 2013 update to the American Psychiatric Association's classifications and diagnoses of mental disorders. Treatment recommendations as well as health insurance payment guidelines are included in the *DSM-V*.

In addition, the *DSM-V* is aligned with the eleventh edition of the WHO's *International Classification of Diseases*. This international reference tome assists mental health professionals with consistent communications about symptoms and severity of depression.

These august references explain that potential depressive symptoms are somewhat common, and by themselves are not indicative of depression. However, the *DSM-V* states that five or more of the following symptoms that occur nearly *daily* during the same two-week period are attributable to a depression diagnosis:

* Feelings of worthlessness, guilt, helplessness, or hopelessness.
* Loss of interest in previously enjoyed activities.
* Exhibiting a pessimistic attitude or outlook.
* Thoughts of death or suicide.
* Sleep issues, early awakening, or oversleeping.
* Decreased energy or fatigue.
* Irritability or restlessness.
* Difficulty concentrating or making decisions.
* Low appetite or overeating.

* Persistent sadness, anxiety, or a feeling of emptiness.

One of my depressive symptoms was crying over nothing. During my more severe bouts of depression, I could look at a blank wall and begin crying. I also would cry over deaths of celebrities for whom I had no particular affinity.

Another depressive symptom is having persistent physical symptoms such as headaches, digestive issues, and pain for which no physical cause can be diagnosed. For example, researchers from Rice University learned that depression is connected to chronic inflammation. This study, published in a 2017 issue of *Psychoneuroendocrinology*, examined the mental and physical health of 1,085 participants, 56 percent of whom were female. The research team concluded that 1) depression creates an immune system response, and 2) there is a link between depression and heart disease.

Unfortunately, I have experienced all of the abovementioned symptoms. Fortunately, after treatment, I rarely experience any of my previous symptoms.

In the next chapter we will take a look at several common myths and truths about depression.

Chapter 3

Depression Myths and Truths

Since the centuries-long stigma of depression still pervades today, I think it's a good idea to look at common myths and corresponding facts about this condition.

Myth: Depression is caused by a personal weakness.
Truth: Depression is *not* a character flaw. As *Silent Inheritance* explains, depression is most likely caused by genetic variants (or single

nucleotide polymorphisms, SNPs) switched on by environmental or epigenetic factors.

Myth: People with depression never get better.
Truth: With the right treatment, depressed people indeed recover and lead healthy and satisfying lives. I am living proof of recovery from depression! And it's a wonderful feeling!

Myth: People with depression should be institutionalized.
Truth: This perception began in the 1800s, when mentally ill patients were admitted to asylums, hospitals for psychiatrically disturbed people. The practice gradually fell by the wayside during the twentieth century. Nonetheless, some mentally ill people were still hospitalized in "clinics" or "units." In the twenty-first century, most people with depression are not institutionalized, thanks to modern medicine as well as talk therapy.

Myth: Depressed people can control their behavior.
Truth: Most people with depression who understand their symptoms can successfully control their behavior with conventional medication. Please keep in mind that medications may not be 100 percent effective, but they usually do reduce the symptoms and the length of time when behavior can go awry.

Myth: Treatment of depression, when compared to other physical conditions, is below par.
Truth: This is true. Lack of access to professional help as well as quality of treatment for depression has become an issue, at least for Americans.

According to findings published in the April 2017 issue of the journal *Psychiatric Services*, more Americans are suffering from mental health issues including depression, yet many go without proper treatment. Lead author Dr. Judith Weissman, an epidemiologist at NYU's Langone Medical Center, explained, "Mental illness doesn't have parity with physical illness. When a person goes in to get their blood pressure checked, they need to be screened for depression, anxiety, and suicidal ideation. Mental illness needs to be viewed as something as serious as having a stroke or cancer."

Thankfully, there is hope for us. Dr. Weissman stressed, "There's a lot of hope. When you feel like there's no hope, just understand that's the mental illness talking. You can feel better."

Exactly. When you are not feeling mentally well, your neurotransmitters are out of balance. Medication and appropriate diet can make you feel better. I am the living truth, and hope you will be, too.

In the next chapter we will take a brief look at an important biochemical process called methylation that is relevant to depression.

Chapter 4

Introduction to Methylation

More than three billion times a second, a biochemical process called *methylation* cycles throughout the seventy-five trillion cells in your body. In less than a blink of an eye, methylation influences myriad critical functions in your body, including DNA gene expression, thinking, behavior, production and metabolism of neurotransmitters, and manufacturing energy. Without methylation, we would die.

At least one in every two persons is estimated to have at least one gene variant, or SNP, in the methylation cycle. With insufficient functioning of methylation, our mental health may be compromised.

GEEK SPEAK: Methylation occurs when a methyl group (CH_3) bonds with an enzyme to perform a specific action.

As the term methylation suggests, specific enzymes need to hitch a ride with a methyl group called a methyl donor. In order for methylation to work properly, methyl donors, including methionine and SAMe, must initiate the methylation process with homocysteine, a building-block protein.

The Four Cycles of Methylation

Methylation encompasses four concurrent cycles: methionine, folate, BH4, and urea. When I think about methylation, I picture four circles, each representing a cycle, and each connecting at one point with the next circle. Think of cogs in a wheel, going around and around. This is important because some genes hand off their responsibilities to other genes in the adjacent circle.

When we think of methyl groups attaching themselves to genes in the methylation cycle in order to methylate, is it possible to methylate too much or too little?

The answer is yes. Methylation, like most biochemical processes, is about equilibrium. I believe that one is not necessarily an under- or overmethylator for life. There are many symptoms and traits for each one type. And please keep in mind that some people enjoy smooth methylation, i.e., they have no significant methylation gene variants, or unexpressed (not turned on by epigenetics) methylation-related gene mutations.

Ascertaining your histamine level is key to diagnosing over- and undermethylation. Simply stated, low whole-blood histamine and absolute basophils (a type of white blood cell) are indicators of overmethylation. Conversely, an overload of whole-blood histamine (greater than 70 ng/mL) and high absolute basophils (over 1 percent) indicate undermethylation. A blood test is required to obtain these measurements.

An easy way to remember these concepts is to think in the opposite way: LOW histamine and basophils may equate to OVERmethylation. And HIGH histamine and basophils may indicate UNDERmethylation.

Undermethylation

A pioneer in mental health disorders and nutrition, William J. Walsh, PhD, stated in his book *Nutrient Power* that about 38 percent of individuals in his depression database (of about three thousand patients) "exhibit undermethylation as their dominant chemical imbalance." Undermethylators have reduced serotonin, dopamine, and norepinephrine, and are sensitive to the methyl/folate ratio in the brain.

Methyl and folate have opposite epigenetic effects on the expression of neurotransmitter transporters that control synaptic activity in the brain. For example, Dr. Walsh states that "an abnormally low methyl/folate ratio is associated with low levels of serotonin, dopamine, and norepinephrine at brain synapses."

Undermethylation does not equate to under-supplementation. Based on data from hundreds of undermethylated depressive patients, Dr. Walsh cautioned that "folates, choline, manganese, copper…tend to *worsen* their depression and must be strictly avoided." In particular, folate and choline can increase serotonin levels.

Dr. Walsh advises supplementation with SAMe (S-adenosylmethionine) or methionine as potential treatment for undermethylators. Other nutrients, including tryptophan, vitamin B6, vitamin C, and 5-HTP, may be helpful to undermethylators, but check first with your doctor, especially if you are taking prescription antidepressants. If you do decide to supplement with any of these nutrients, start slowly by taking a starting dose of only one supplement (preferably not a multi-supplement) and see if your symptoms improve. My personal opinion for undermethylators is to keep supplementation to a minimum, if at all.

According to Dr. Walsh, undermethylated depressive patients present at least some of these symptoms and traits:

* Obsessive-compulsive tendencies
* History of perfectionism
* Social isolation
* History of high competitiveness
* Self-motivated during school
* Seasonal inhalant allergies
* High inner tension
* Addictive tendencies
* Strong-willed
* History of high accomplishment, both personal and family
* Positive response to SSRIs and antihistamines.

Methylation SNPs, if expressed, can contribute to undermethylation; they include *MTHFR C677T*, *MTHFR A1298C*, *BHMT*, *MAT*, *MS*, and *SAHH*.

When I first unearthed these common symptoms and traits, I was surprised to see myself, all the way back to the beginning of school at age five. In fact, my first-grade teacher emphatically told my mother during her first-ever parent–teacher conference that I was a "perfectionist." Who knew?

Overmethylation

Approximately 20 percent of Dr. Walsh's depressive individuals in his database are overmethylators. These people are generally low in histamine and folate. Remember that low whole-blood histamine (lower than 40 ng/mL) and a low absolute basophil count below 30 indicate potential overmethylation.

Overmethylated depressive persons, according to Dr. Walsh, exhibit symptoms and traits including:

* High anxiety and panic tendency
* Food and chemical sensitivities
* Nervous legs, pacing
* Noncompetitive in sports and games
* Underachievement in school
* Estrogen intolerance
* Adverse response to SSRIs and antihistamines
* Low motivation
* Excess body hair
* Absence of seasonal inhalant allergies
* Artistic or music ability

Single nucleotide polymorphisms associated with overmethylation include: *CBS, GAMT, AGAT, and MT.*

As expected, I do not have these symptoms and traits because I am an undermethylator. But can we swing in either direction? After all, our methylation whirls within us at the mind-boggling rate of billions of times per second. Is it possible to have traits of both under- and overmethylation? I believe so.

In the next chapter let's look at how methylation affects your thinking and behavior—the importance of specific neurotransmitters: serotonin, dopamine, and norepinephrine.

Chapter 5

Neurotransmitters

Neurotransmitters are brain chemicals that are responsible for your thinking, mood, emotions, memory, energy, libido, cravings, and sleep. They are produced in the roughly eighty-six billion neurons (nerve cells) housed in the brain. Think of neurotransmitters as chemical messengers communicating smoothly with one another so our brain operates normally. When specific neurotransmitters are out of sync, we can feel depressed.

Having researched how neurotransmitters work in the brain, I have decided to spare you the technical and medical language as much as possible. The most important thing to know is that neurotransmitters must be balanced; if they are not, depression symptoms can occur. Silent inheritance of mutations in expressed genes essential to the production of neurotransmitters may cause this imbalance.

Let's look at three primary neurotransmitters that are related to depression: serotonin, dopamine, and norepinephrine.

Serotonin

Serotonin is the king of the depression-related neurotransmitters. It influences the brain cells related to, inter alia, mood, sexual desire and function, sleep, and some types of social behavior. When serotonin levels are balanced, they enhance the feelings of peace, joy, calm, and gratitude.

Although serotonin is produced in the brain, about 90 percent of the serotonin supply is located in the digestive tract and blood platelets. This fact accentuates the importance of a healthy gut (see chapter 9).

The methylation process is directly involved in the production of serotonin, where production begins with an amino acid called tryptophan. When tryptophan is combined with another amino acid called 5-hydroxytryptamine (5-HTP), they rely on a compound called BH4, which requires active folate (5-MTHF) from the folate cycle and SAMe from the methionine cycle. The end result is serotonin.

As part of the methylation process, serotonin is broken down by the monoamine oxidase type A (*MAO-A*) gene into ammonia and other detoxification products. However, when you have a positive *MAO-A* mutation, the detoxification process may be imbalanced and cause fatigue and brain fog.

Furthermore, the *MAO-A* gene variant is associated with depression, anxiety, and other mood disorders. The biochemical imbalance of serotonin levels may be a result of a shortage of tryptophan, low neuronal production of serotonin, a reduced level of serotonin receptor sites, or the inability of serotonin to attach to receptor sites.

Dopamine

The neurotransmitter dopamine helps control the brain's reward and pleasure centers. It also assists with regulation of movement and emotional responses. Similar to serotonin, dopamine is made in the brain and is replete in the gut.

Symptoms of low dopamine include: low mood, difficulty getting motivated, and feelings of worthlessness and hopelessness. People who have low dopamine tend to be noncompliant, potentially being difficult to treat with nutritional protocols and antidepressants.

It is common to see persons with both low serotonin and dopamine. These patients may need treatments for the diminished levels of both neurotransmitters. For example, a patient could take both a selective serotonin reuptake inhibitor (SSRI) and a norepinephrine dopamine reuptake inhibitor (NDRI). (Please see chapter 13 for additional information.)

The methylation process is also directly involved in the production of dopamine, where production begins with an amino acid called tyrosine. Tyrosine relies on a compound called BH4, which requires 5-MTHF from the folate cycle and SAMe from the methionine cycle. The end result is dopamine.

Norepinephrine

As the methylation child of dopamine, norepinephrine (noradrenaline), when released, has an impact on the "fight-or-flight" stress response. Regarding depression, norepinephrine is involved in mood, emotions, and behavior.

People with low norepinephrine may experience lethargy, brain fog, and lack of enthusiasm for life. It is common to see people taking antidepressants that include a norepinephrine reuptake inhibitor.

Norepinephrine is produced in the brain, central nervous system, and adrenal glands. This neurotransmitter, like serotonin and dopamine, can be found in the gastrointestinal tract.

In the next chapter we look at gene variants that are related to depression.

Chapter 6

Depression-Related Gene Variants

Let's look at a brief overview of what DNA looks like and how it can change, creating a gene variant. Please remember that carrying any of the single nucleotide polymorphisms (SNPs) or gene variants does not mean that you will have symptoms of depression. However, depression-related SNPs that are turned on by epigenetics may present depression symptoms.

> GEEK SPEAK: Each DNA base pair, e.g., AT or CG, has a sugar molecule and a phosphate molecule attached to it. These three components create a nucleotide. Nucleotides form in two long spiral strands—a double helix—that resembles a ladder. Base pairs are the rungs; the sugar and phosphate molecules form the vertical sides of the ladder.

MTHFR Gene Variants

"I have the *MTHFR* mutation," emphatically stated a member of my social media Vitamin D Wellness group. "What should I do?" she inquired.

Having read thousands of posts, mostly related to vitamin D, on the group's page, I realized the member's comment was a first for me. I had no idea what she was talking about! "*MTHFR*"—what is that? Intellectual curiosity and the desire to help group members prompted me to begin a journey that led me to writing *Silent Inheritance*.

First, I learned that *MTHFR* refers to the "methylene tetrahydrofolate reductase" gene that is vital to the smooth process of methylation. Second, I ascertained that there is more than one *MTHFR* mutation. Third, I discovered that methylation-related gene mutations are related to depression.

Before I discuss these gene mutations, I should explain the words "heterozygous" and "homozygous." Heterozygous means that the gene mutation has one copy from one of your biological parents. Homozygous means that the gene mutation has two copies, one from each of your biological parents.

Being heterozygous is not as potentially severe as being homozygous. For example, a woman with homozygous *MTHFR C677T* inherited one copy of the gene variant from her biological father and one from her biological mother. This female may endure methylation that is only performing at 30 percent. If she had been heterozygous for *MTHFR C677T*, her methylation cycle may perform much better—around 70 percent.

MTHFR C677T Gene Variant

Regarding the relationship between methylation and depression, there are two primary gene variants: *MTHFR C677T* (rs1801133) and *MTHFR A1298C* (rs1801131). The *MTHFR C677T* gene variant is the more common of the two. (Please note that each SNP is assigned an "rs" or "reference SNP" number by the US National Center for Biotechnology Information.)

About 57 percent of the global population carries at least one copy of the *MTHFR C677T* mutation. Not surprisingly, I am heterozygous *MTHFR C677T*—no doubt a contributor to my depression.

MTHFR A1298C Gene Variant

The *MTHFR A1298C* gene variant may increase the risk of developing depression. The *MTHFR*

A1298C SNP slows the body down to make BH4, which is essential to produce neurotransmitters including serotonin, dopamine, and norepinephrine.

About 23 percent of the world's population has the *MTHFR A1298C* SNP. I tested negative for *MTHFR A1298C*.

MAO-A Gene Variants

The monoamine oxidase A (*MAO-A*) gene is commonly referred to as the "warrior gene," owing to its association with aggression in some people. In 1993, the *MAO-A* gene was first linked to antisocial behavior when it was identified in a large Dutch family that was infamous for violence. The nickname "warrior gene" was coined at the 2004 annual meeting of the American Association of Physical Anthropologists, according to a piece published in the journal *Science*.

The *MAO-A* gene in the BH4 methylation cycle is directly associated with depression. *MAO-A* breaks down serotonin, dopamine, and norepinephrine. The rapid degradation of these neurotransmitters is crucial to smooth functioning during synaptic transmission in the central nervous system.

A variant in the *MAO-A R297R* (rs6323) gene may decrease the metabolism of serotonin, dopamine, and norepinephrine, resulting in higher levels of these neurotransmitters and lower levels of their respective metabolites. The *MAO-A* gene also is associated with obsessive-compulsive disorder (OCD), anxiety, and a host of other brain conditions.

At least one-third of the population carries the *MAO-A* gene mutation. I am homozygous for the *MAO-A R297R* (rs6323). In addition, the scientific community has identified at least two other depression-related *MAO-A* gene variants: rs3027399 and rs909525. I am negative for *MAO-A* rs3027399 and heterozygous for *MAO-A* rs909525.

COMT Gene Variants

The catechol-O-methyltransferase (*COMT*) genes interact with the MAO-A genes. Like the MAO-A genes, the *COMT* genes work in the BH4 cycle of methylation.

COMT genes are primarily responsible for breaking down dopamine and adrenaline (epinephrine). Moreover, *COMT* genes are players in the breakdown of estrogen in the liver.

Approximately 59 percent of the world's population carries the *COMT* (rs6269) SNP, according to LiveWello, a software interpretation service. The only *COMT* SNP that I was positive for is the *COMT* rs6269. I am negative for *COMT* *V158M* (rs4680), *COMT* *H62H* (rs4633), and *COMT* *P199P* (rs769224). Since I am homozygous for both *MAO-A R297R* (rs6323) and *COMT* rs6269, I am at an increased risk of depression, and certainly have experienced the symptoms.

DAO Gene Variants

Scientific research indicates that variants in D-amino acid oxidase (*DAO*) genes (rs3741775 and rs2070586) are primarily related to schizophrenia and bipolar affective disorder. However, I think they may also affect depression. *DAO* enzymes affect the degradation of histamine. When this process is inhibited by a turned-on *DAO* variant, dopamine synthesis may be compromised. This potential action makes sense to me because I am homozygous for *DAO* (rs3741775), and I am being treated for dopamine balancing.

According to the LiveWello website, about half of the global population has the *DAO* rs3741775 SNP. I am homozygous for *DAO* (rs3741775) gene variant and have no copies of *DAO* rs2070586.

VDR Gene Variants

Vitamin D deficiency is rampant around the globe. Modern lifestyles and decades-long admonitions from the medical community often deny us the most natural source of vitamin D: the sun. Moreover, we may be born with a genetic predisposition to poorly metabolize vitamin D.

Two common vitamin-D-related gene variants are *VDR Taq* and *VDR Bsm*. The *VDR* SNPs adversely affect depression because they mediate the production of the neurotransmitter dopamine.

More than one-fourth of the world's population has inherited at least one of these two gene variants that are related to vitamin D metabolism.

I inherited the *VDR Taq* (+/-) from one parent and the *VDR Bsm* (+/-) SNPs from one parent. Anyone who has inherited these homozygous (+/+) *VDR* gene polymorphisms from both biological parents may experience not only a vitamin D deficiency but medical conditions associated with low vitamin D. (Please see chapter 11 for additional information about vitamin D.)

GAD1 Gene Variants

The glutamate decarboxylase 1 (*GAD1*) gene variants are perhaps lesser known as depression-related SNPs than the aforementioned gene mutations in this chapter. Vitamin B6 is a cofactor to the *GAD1* genes that convert glutamate to gamma-aminobutyric acid (GABA), a "downer" neurotransmitter.

Only about 21 percent of the global population has *GAD* rs769407. I am heterozygous for a number of *GAD1* gene variants, including rs769407.

Identification of New Depression-Related Gene Variants

In 2016, US research scientists announced the discovery of fifteen new gene variants associated with depression. Their study, published in the journal *Nature Genetics*, analyzed genetic variants of 75,607 individuals of European ancestry who self-reported depression and 213,747 healthy controls. All participants consented to use their 23andMe data (anonymously) for this research.

The following depression-related SNPs were discovered as a result of the research explained above:

rs10514299	*TMEM161B-MEF2C*
rs454214	*TMEM161B-MEF2C*
rs1518395	*VRK2*
rs2179744	*L3MBTL2*
rs11209948	*NEGR1*
rs2422321	*NEGR1*
rs301806	*RERE*
rs1475120	*HACE1-LIN28B*
rs10786831	*SORCS3*
rs12552	*OLFM4*
rs6476606	*PAX5*
rs8025231	*MEIS2-TMCO5A*
rs1656369	*RSRC1-MLF1*
rs2125716	*SLC6A15*
rs7044150	*KIAA0020-RFX3*

These SNPs are included in the dbSNP database, a free public archive for genetic variation within and across different species, developed and hosted by the National Center for Biotechnology Information in collaboration with the National Human Genome Research Institute.

At the time of this writing, not all of these SNPs are included in the 23andMe and Ancestry raw data from the saliva sample.

In the next chapter I explain the types of available genetic and neurotransmitter tests.

Chapter 7

Genetic and Neurotransmitter Testing

I n this chapter I address how to test your DNA single nucleotide polymorphisms (SNPs) and neurotransmitters. You can find out your genetic predisposition to neurotransmitter imbalances by taking a relatively affordable saliva test at home. Some urine and blood tests are also available.

Saliva Testing

Thanks to the 2003 completion of the Human Genome Study, the accessibility of genetic testing has transformed from a test for only the wealthy to being relatively inexpensive, starting at USD$99 at the time of this writing. Moreover, a genetic test kit is easily obtainable online and done in the privacy of your home.

Please understand that results of saliva testing yield genetic predispositions. They tell us what genes have been mutated, possibly affecting your neurotransmitter balance. In the next chapter I will show you how to interpret your depression-related genetic saliva test data.

Ancestry DNA Test

Are you one of the two million members of Ancestry.com? If you have taken Ancestry's DNA saliva test to ascertain your ethnic heritage, you can easily obtain some of the key genetic mutations data related to depression including *MTHFR*, *COMT*, *VDR*, and *MAO* SNPs for free!

At the time of this writing, the Ancestry DNA test is available to residents of the United

States, Canada, United Kingdom, Australia, New Zealand, South Korea, Ireland, the Netherlands, Denmark, Finland, and Sweden as well as about twenty other European countries.

If you want to take Ancestry's DNA saliva test, check out the Ancestry.com website. At the time of this writing, the cost of the DNA saliva test is USD$99.

Once you have your raw DNA data from Ancestry.com, simply download the data and upload them to GeneticGenie.org to find out a limited number of your SNPs. The use of GeneticGenie.org is free of charge, but donations are gratefully accepted.

23andMe Test

Until about September 2017, the most comprehensive SNP test available to the general public was obtained from 23andMe.com. For about USD$99, you received genetic data, which included your methylation SNPs.

Unfortunately, 23andMe modified the gene variants to be tested and excluded the warrior gene *MAO-A* as well as other methylation SNPs. Based on this change, I do not recommend 23andMe testing if you are interested in the SNPs related to methylation and depression.

Personally, I have used both Ancestry and 23andMe. I found Ancestry's data to be sufficient when examining methylation profile SNPs that affect the balance of neurotransmitters.

LabCorp

Another noninvasive test for *MTHFR* only is LabCorp's (a popular laboratory in the United States) buccal swab test. Buccal swab means that you collect *MTHFR* DNA from the cells on the inside of the cheeks. This type of DNA testing is good for babies, young children, and other people who may have difficulty spitting in a tube for several minutes.

Urine Testing

Labrix Clinical Services, Inc. offers a simple urine test that reports levels of neurotransmitters including serotonin, dopamine, and norepinephrine. The great aspect about this test is that it is much easier to interpret than the genetic tests results. The test report depicts the measurement of each neurotransmitter on a reference range scale and provides an interpretation of the results.

The Labrix Neurotransmitter Test is available through medical professionals who are providers of this service. The test kit (about USD$191) is also available from Amazon and canaryclub.org. According to Labrix, the test kit is available to residents of most countries.

In addition, LabCorp conducts a whole-blood test on *MTHFR C677T* and *MTHFR A1298C*. Another well-known lab called Quest Diagnostics also provides blood testing of these two *MTHFR* gene variants.

Blood Testing

MTHFR Testing

The SpectraCell MTHFR Genetic Test identifies two of the most common mutations that occur in the methylation cycle: *MTHFR C677T* and *MTHFR A1298C*. You may recall the importance of these genotypes in methylation from chapter 4.

The SpectraCell test is useful only if you want to know about your *MTHFR* status. Unlike the genetic saliva tests, only two gene variants are analyzed. For the approximate cost of USD$150, blood is collected in a medical practitioner's office and analyzed by SpectraCell's accredited laboratory. (Please note that to order the test your physician must be a SpectraCell provider.)

The popular LabCorp conducts a whole-blood test on *MTHFR C677T* and *MTHFR A1298C*. The cost of the test depends on your health-care insurance.

Another well-known lab called Quest Diagnostics also provides blood testing for both primary *MTHFR* SNPs. Once again, cost of this test is dependent on your medical insurance.

Histamine Testing

Remember when we discussed over- and undermethylation and their relationship to depression in chapter 4? You may recall the positive relationship between the neurotransmitter histamine and depression.

High histamine equates to undermethylators, who often suffer from, inter alia, depression and obsessive-compulsive disorder (OCD). People with low histamine are overmethylators and typically may endure anxiety, panic attacks, and paranoia.

In addition to assessing methylation symptoms, it is useful to test whole-blood histamine in your medical practitioner's office. This test is an evaluation of the level of histamine to ascertain whether you are under- or overmethylating. Generally speaking, many insurance plans cover the cost of the approximately USD$80 blood test.

Chapter 8 explains how to read DNA testing results using GeneticGenie. org.

Figure 1: Author's Methylation Profile

genetic genie

Profile: Methylation Profile
Generated: 8/6/2017

Gene & Variation	rsID	Alleles	Result
COMT V158M	rs4680	GG	-/-
COMT H62H	rs4633	CC	-/-
COMT P199P	rs769224	GG	-/-
VDR Bsm	rs1544410	CT	+/-
VDR Taq	rs731236	AG	+/-
MAO A R297R	rs6323	TT	+/+
ACAT1-02	rs3741049	GG	-/-
MTHFR C677T	rs1801133	AG	+/-
MTHFR 03 P39P	rs2066470	GG	-/-
MTHFR A1298C	rs1801131	TT	-/-
MTR A2756G	rs1805087	AA	-/-
MTRR A66G	rs1801394	GG	+/+
MTRR H595Y	not found	n/a	not genotyped
MTRR K350A	rs162036	AA	-/-
MTRR R415T	not found	n/a	not genotyped
MTRR A664A	rs1802059	GG	-/-
BHMT-02	rs567754	CT	+/-
BHMT-04	not found	n/a	not genotyped
BHMT-08	rs651852	TT	+/+
AHCY-01	rs819147	CT	+/-
AHCY-02	not found	n/a	not genotyped
AHCY-19	rs819171	CT	+/-
CBS C699T	rs234706	AG	+/-
CBS A360A	rs1801181	GG	-/-
CBS N212N	not found	n/a	not genotyped
SHMT1 C1420T	not found	n/a	not genotyped

Chapter 8

Understanding Genetic
Test Results

When you receive your DNA test results, how do you know if you are predisposed to depression? An example of a methylation profile results page, generated by GeneticGenie. org, is contained in Figure 1.

The left-most column lists the genes and their variants, e.g., *COMT V158M*. Each line corresponds to a SNP or gene variant.

The second column contains the rsID assigned to a particular SNP. For example, the rsID for the *COMT V158M* gene variant is rs4680. Remember that "rs" or "reference SNP" numbers are assigned in accession by the US National Center for Biotechnology Information.

The third column contains the alleles for the DNA base pairs. For example, the paired alleles "GG" represent one of each of the two chromosome pairs. An allele is a variant form of a gene that is formulated by a mutation.

The far-right column states the result for a particular SNP. The possibilities are -/- or negative; +/- or positive for one copy from a biological parent, also called "heterozygous"; and +/+ or positive with two copies of the gene mutation, one from each biological parent, also called "homozygous." The result of *COMT V158M* in Figure 1 indicates that the individual (genotype) is -/- for *COMT V158M*.

You will note that in some cases "not genotyped" is stated as a result. This simply means that the SNP is not available in the pool of data used by 23andMe, Ancestry, or another genetic testing service.

A Look at My Genotype

By using 23andMe data in Figure 1, we can analyze my genotype for methylation. I am only +/+ or homozygous for three SNPs: *MAO-A R297R*, *MTRR A66G*, and *BHMT-08*. I am +/- or heterozygous for both *VDR Bsm* and *VDR Taq*, *MTHFR C677T*, *BHMT-02*, *AHCY-01*, *AHCY-19*, and *CBS C699T*. The remainder of the listed SNPs are negative, normal, or "not genotyped."

So, regarding depression, what does my methylation profile indicate about me?

1) I am heterozygous for *MTHFR C677T*. A relationship between *MTHFR C677T* and depressive symptoms has been established.

2) I am homozygous for *MAO-A R297R*, the "warrior" gene. This gene variant, when

expressed, may diminish the metabolism of serotonin, dopamine, and norepineph-rine, resulting in an imbalance of these neurotransmitters.

3) I am heterozygous for both *VDR* SNPs, which mediate the production of do-pamine, potentially causing uneven amounts of this neurotransmitter.

In addition, I have other depression-related SNPs from running my data through other genetic reporting services like LiveWello. Unfortunately, the software used by various genetic reporting entities clearly varies. For example, LiveWello reports my *MAO-A R297R* as negative, yet the raw data processed by 23and-dMe and Ancestry indicate that I am homozy-gous! I wish I had an answer to this issue, and hope that the accuracy of genetic reporting will improve.

Let's look at epigenetics to learn what causes gene variants to turn on.

Chapter 9

Epigenetic Influences on Gene Variants

Throughout *Silent Inheritance* I mention the impact of stressors in your life that may negatively influence the expression of your inherited gene variants. What this means is that epigenetic, or environmental, stress may cause gene variants to become expressed or to "turn on."

A few truths to keep in mind before discussing epigenetics:

1) Every individual differs biochemically and genetically.
2) Every person perceives stress differently, and reacts to stress in one's own unique way.
3) A treatment, natural or conventional, that works for one individual may not work in the same way for another person.

Remember that your gene variants have been passed down over scores of generations. For example, my genetic makeup has been traced back to over 275,000 years ago!

It is important *not* to blame living biological relatives for your *silent inheritance* of depression-related gene variants. Chances are highly likely that your genes mutated over many centuries. Simply put, your inherited depression is not anyone's fault!

The best thing to do is to accept your gene variants, learn about them, and develop a plan to minimize the likelihood of them turning on.

And if your gene variants are expressed symptomatically, develop a strategy to diminish any negative effects.

As you read this book, think of what surrounds you: the air you breathe, the materials of the indoor space where you might be sitting, the food and beverages you consumed today, the cosmetics you are wearing, and the medicines you are taking. We are hard-pressed to avoid contaminated environments, as they are so widespread in everyday life. In addition, think of life-related stress that you have experienced over years or decades.

Environmental Pollutants

Let's first look at the air we breathe indoors. The number of chemicals that lurk in your household surroundings is daunting. Household products including furniture, mattresses, building materials, cabinets, wallpaper, and cleaning products are capable of "off-gassing" or emitting gases into your indoor air. Inside pollutants capable of disrupting your DNA are flame retardants and formaldehyde.

Combine the outdoor air pollution in your area (outdoor pollution is common in developed areas and varies day-to-day) with the indoor pollution, and you can see the prevalence of air pollution in our lives.

Another class of environmental culprits is called volatile organic compounds, or VOCs. These VOCs encompass a vast family of chemicals that contain carbon and hydrogen. Using aerosol sprays only exacerbates the dissemination of these inhaled chemicals. They can be released in the air via tobacco smoke, vehicle exhaust, and personal care products.

Did you know there are about 4,800 chemicals in cigarette smoke, many of which are capable of damaging DNA? And one puff of smoke may contain 10 trillion free radicals, according to a 2013 study by an Indian research team.

Whether it is your hair, nails, or makeup, the list of product contaminants in shampoo, hairspray, nail varnish, perfume, body lotion, lipstick, deodorant, foundation, blush, and eye shadow is long. Remember that what you apply to your face is absorbed by your body and could disrupt your gene variants!

Food and Beverage Consumption

Much of the food we consume contains chemicals that may adversely affect our bodies. In fact, research has shown an association between the brain, the gut, and depression. Gut microorganisms, capable of producing and delivering neurotransmitters, can activate immune and neuroendocrine systems in the gastrointestinal tract.

Furthermore, food exposed to chemicals may contribute to mitochondrial dysfunction, also connected to depression. The cells' energy stores are called mitochondria, found in every cell of your body except for the red blood cells.

Many retail stores are laden with genetically modified organism (GMO) foods. GMO foods are a result of "foreign genes" artificially forced into the natural genes of another type of plant or animal. Assume that such nonorganic foods are laced with toxic pesticides.

An organophosphate chemical compound called glyphosate is an herbicide that is applied to fruits, vegetables, grains, and meats. Ingesting these tainted nonorganic foods might adversely affect gene variants, potentially contributing to depressive symptoms. My literature research surprisingly (or not) revealed that the ear tags attached to animals contain pesticides.

Another concern is folic acid. If you carefully check the ingredient labels on processed foods, you probably will see "folic acid" added to at least some of them. As you know from a basic understanding of methylation, folic acid is synthetic and unrecognized by the methionine methylation cycle. Folic acid is yet another potential gene disruptor.

Consuming alcohol is another potential way of expressing gene variants. By metabolizing alcohol, a chemical called acetaldehyde is formed. This process generates a large number of free radicals that wreak havoc, causing oxidative stress. Oxidative stress is generated by epigenetic factors and may influence by turning on gene variants.

Sugar is another "bad actor" when it comes to increasing the risk of depression. A July 2017 study, published in *Scientific Reports*, discovered that over a five-year period, men with the highest sugar intake from foods and beverages had a 23 percent increase in their risk of developing mental health issues including depression. Beware of consuming any types of added sugars.

Common over-the-counter and prescription medications may contribute to nutritional deficiencies. For example, metformin, a popular medicine prescribed to treat diabetes, may deplete B vitamins and vitamin D3. Over-the-counter NSAIDs also decrease the nutritional value of these vitamins.

Life-Related Stress

Do you recall experiencing stress when you were a child? How about as a teenager? An adult? Stress might be related to relationships, work, health, and money. Most of us have endured lots of stress from these factors.

I believe my depression is directly associated with life-related stress. As a young child beginning school, I was scared and conflicted. I loved doing schoolwork but I felt uneasy, gawky, and less than confident. I was bullied every school day for years—by girls my own age.

Once I entered high school, I gained significant self-confidence and focused on pursuing friendships and college education. I loved every minute of my undergraduate days, and later enjoyed a successful but stressful career. So, what was the source of stress over decades of my life? Being a perfectionist. (Yes, my first-grade teacher was absolutely correct!) I also was highly competitive and felt constant pressure to perform my best as a woman working in a man's world.

Any of these epigenetic factors may ignite inflammation, culminating in stress and the expression of gene variants. Some of these epigenetic factors are difficult to escape, so what can you do to avoid turning on your depression-related gene variants?

The bottom-line answer is to maintain a healthy lifestyle:

* Consume organic foods and beverages; eschew sugars and folic acid in your diet.
* Avoid alcohol intake.
* Refrain from smoking.
* Exercise at least twenty minutes, three times a week.
* Avoid cosmetic aerosols such as hair and deodorant sprays.
* Make time for yourself; meditate.

* Supplement with vitamin D3, vitamin K2, and magnesium.
* Consider taking folate, B6, and B12 in accordance with your medication as well as the information contained in the next chapter.

Chapter 10

The Big Three B Vitamins

A smoothly run methylation cycle contributes to diminishing depression symptoms. The proper balance of folate, vitamin B6, and vitamin B12 is paramount to healthy methylation.

The relationship between folate, vitamin B6, and vitamin B12 and depression has been examined for decades. More recently, a team of Canadian researchers led by Laura Gougeon, PhD, studied the effect of dietary intake of folate, vitamin B6, and vitamin B12 on older adults (67–83 years old) to ascertain the risk of depression from them. These studies, published in a 2016 issue of the *European Journal of Clinical Nutrition* and a 2017 edition of the *British Journal of Nutrition*, suggest an association between folate, vitamin B6, and vitamin B12 and depression risk. For example, depressed individuals had consistently lower dietary intakes of these three B nutrients.

Let's look individually at these three water-soluble nutrients. How do they relate to depression? What foods and supplements could fortify you with these vitamins? When should you not take these vitamins? How can you test for levels of the "Big Three?"

Folate

Folate is actually vitamin B9, and is often confused with the synthetic "folic acid." People with *MTHFR* gene variants should avoid folic acid. Moreover, I think everyone should avoid folic acid, as it is synthetic and can disrupt methylation.

Unfortunately, many processed foods contain folic acid. I always suggest reading ingredient labels on food products as well as supplements to avoid folic acid as much as possible.

In addition, please note that "folic acid" and "folinic acid" are not the same. Folic acid is synthetic, and folinic acid is a form of folate found naturally in food.

Folate is involved in the biosynthesis of the neurotransmitters including serotonin and dopamine. If folate levels are too low, serotonin and dopamine can decrease, adversely affecting mood and motivation.

Dietary Intake. Foods rich in folate include spinach, some legumes, asparagus, romaine lettuce, sunflower seeds, avocado, broccoli, and oranges.

Supplementation. Regarding supplementing with folate, ensure that folic acid is not an ingredient. If it is, place the product back on the shelf. Overall, L-methyl-folate is the correct supplement, but first, please see the "To Methylate or Not" section at the end of this chapter. Start slow with a folate supplement that contains 200 mcg. Another folate "supplement" is Deplin (7.5 mg), which is only available by prescription, at least in the United States.

Testing. The most reliable test for folate is called "RBC folate." When I requested this blood test, I received results for *serum folic acid*, a waste of my money and time. I can't emphasize enough to get the *folate* in your *red blood cells* (RBC) tested. The RBC folate reference range for adults is 140–628 ng/mL (317–1422 nmol/L); for children, over 160 ng/mL (362 nmol/L).

Histamine is another indicator of folate level. So, another measurement related to folate is to test whole-blood histamine. If the value is lower than 4.0 ng/mL, you may have a folate deficiency.

Vitamin B6

Another common deficiency is vitamin B6. Depression is associated with low levels of vitamin B6, causing dopamine to become imbalanced.

Dietary Intake. Foods containing vitamin B6 include chicken, fish, lean meats, non-citrus fruits, and pistachio nuts.

Supplementation. If you wish to supplement with vitamin B6, P-5-P (pyridoxal-5-phosphate) is the active form, and is readily available at online stores. A conservative starting dose is 25 mg.

Testing. To test vitamin B6, take the blood test called "PLP (pyridoxal phosphate)." The reference range for this test is 5–50 mcg/L.

Vitamin B12

With causes ranging from eating vegan or vegetarian to taking diabetes medications or proton-pump inhibitors, vitamin B12 deficiency is quite common today. In fact, a B12 deficiency may hide under the cloak of symptoms associated with Alzheimer's, dementia, multiple sclerosis, and other serious medical conditions, as symptoms are similar and serum B12 testing is far from accurate.

Vitamin B12 deficiency probably "is not the cause of *most* cases of mental illness, but it clearly plays a powerful role in a number of cases— and particularly in cases involving depression," according to Sally Pacholok and Jeffrey Stuart, coauthors of the popular book entitled *Could It Be B12?* Indeed, vitamin B12 is a vital player in methylation, particularly the synthesis of methionine. This process, of course, leads to neurotransmitter synthesis of serotonin, dopamine, and norepinephrine. Low vitamin B12 can lead to lower levels of these neurotransmitters.

Dietary Intake. Foods rich in B12 include: beef, eggs, fatty fish, oysters, and cottage cheese.

Supplementation. Supplementation with B12 can be tricky, owing to its four forms: cyano-cobalamin, methylcobalamin, adenosylcobala-min, and hydroxocobalamin.

Beware of cyanocobalamin, as it contains a cyanide (yes, the poison) molecule. However, cyanocobalamin is inexpensive and may comprise the contents of a B12 injection. Do not buy cyanocobalamin supplements, and always ask your health-care practitioner what form of B12 a shot (jab) contains before the injection is administrated.

Thankfully, the remaining three forms of B12 supplements are solid options *depending on specific gene variants.* According to Dr. Amy Yasko, vitamin B12 supplementation should be administered according to your *COMT V158M* (rs 4680) and *VDR Taq* (rs 731236) gene variants.

If you are negative (-/-) for *COMT V158M* and positive (+/+ or +/-) for *VDR Taq*, you could tolerate all three forms of B12, taking care with methyl B12 (please see the next section of this chapter).

If you are heterozygous for *COMT V158M* and homozygous for *VDR Taq*, you can tolerate all three types, but with less methyl B12.

If you are heterozygous for *COMT V158M* and heterozygous or negative for *VDR Taq*, you could best tolerate hydroxyl and/or adenosyl B12.

If you are homozygous for *COMT V158M* and homozygous or heterozygous for *VDR Taq*, hydroxyl B12 and/or adenosyl B12 are the best options for you.

If you are homozygous for *COMT V158M* and negative for *VDR Taq*, hydroxyl B12 is the best tolerated form of B12 for you.

I am negative for *COMT V158M* and heterozygous for *VDR Taq*. Therefore, I can tolerate any of the three types of B12. However, I am prudent regarding methyl supplementation (read on).

A conservative starting daily dose of any form of vitamin B12 is 10,000 mcg.

Testing. If you ask for a vitamin B12 test, you most likely will undergo a blood test collection called serum B12. Unfortunately, the serum B12 test does not distinguish between active and inactive B12, calling into question the accuracy of this particular blood test.

A test called MMA (methylmalonic acid) can be conducted using blood or urine. The urinary MMA test is the most accurate method of determining how well your body absorbs vitamin B12. The reference range is 0–0.4 μmol/L.

To Methylate or Not?

As you read in chapter 3, some people under-methylate, and others overmethylate. If you are an overmethylator, refrain from taking methylated supplements. If you are an undermethylator, excess folate tends to worsen depression.

You may have noticed that some B supplements discussed in this chapter have the word "methyl" at the beginning of the supplement name, e.g., methylcobalamin. Since the methylation cycle requires methyl groups in order to function well, it should make sense to take methylated vitamins. However, our methylation cycle can operate under capacity or at a higher-than-normal speed. We aim for the middle—the just-right balance of methylation.

The bottom line is to carefully supplement, with or without added methyl groups—start "low and slow." As an undermethylator, I *occasionally* take one capsule of Dr. Ben Lynch's Seeking Health Homocystex that includes a few methylated B vitamins. I take them in the morning because they provide energy for me.

In the next chapter we'll discuss another supplement, vitamin D3, and its amazing health benefits.

Chapter 11

Vitamin D Wellness

Adequate vitamin D is essential to our health and quality of life. Do you know that every cell in our bodies contains a vitamin D receptor (VDR)? When a VDR is activated by a sufficient intake of vitamin D, good things happen. Vitamin D's mechanisms of action include antimicrobial, anticancer, anti-inflammatory properties. In other words, scientific research indicates that vitamin D deficiency is connected to a wide array of serious medical conditions such as cancer, *depression*, cardiovascular disease, diabetes, as well as multiple sclerosis and other autoimmune diseases.

Due to our modern lifestyles and conventional medical practices, we tend to get little vitamin D from its natural source, the ultraviolet B rays of the sun. From living, commuting, and working indoors to fretfully slapping sunscreen all over our skin, we appear intent on denying ourselves this essential nutrient. As most diets are severely lacking in vitamin D, the most practical way of getting adequate vitamin D is by taking an inexpensive daily oral D3 supplement.

As someone who is impassioned about the health benefits of vitamin D, my vitamin D level has been optimal for years, despite my inherited *VDR* SNPs. Anyone (people with kidney or liver issues should consult their practitioner before supplementation) who has one or more *VDR* gene mutations can overcome this defect by raising one's levels to at least 100 ng/mL (250 nmol/L). In fact, by following my three-nutrient protocol, you most likely will overcome any vitamin-D-related genetic disposition within weeks or a few months.

Vitamin D Wellness Protocol

Tens of thousands of people have accessed my Vitamin D Wellness Protocol on my website, smilinsuepubs.com. Here is the protocol in a nutshell:

Vitamin D: Most diets do not contain adequate vitamin D3. Start by taking 5,000 IU *daily* of vitamin D3 oil-based (soft gels or liquid) supplements with or right after your breakfast. After the first week, take 10,000 IU a day. Enjoy direct noon sun exposure for up to 15–20 minutes a day, when possible.

Vitamin K2: A vitamin K2 diet includes lots of grass-fed meat and dairy products. Since most of us are lacking daily abundant intake of grass-fed goods, consume about 100 mcg of vitamin K2 (MK-7). Take your K2 with your D3 with or right after your breakfast. Please do not take any form of vitamin K if you are on blood-thinning medication without the approval of your health-care practitioner.

Magnesium: Magnesium-rich foods include leafy green vegetables, legumes, nuts, and seeds.

A *daily* supplement of magnesium glycinate (or magnesium citrate if you do not have access to magnesium glycinate) of 400–600 mg should boost your levels of this essential mineral. Take your magnesium glycinate before bedtime. (The glycine in this supplement has a calming effect that should foster sleep.)

Please note that persons taking thyroid medication should wait at least four hours before taking any minerals, including magnesium.

Vitamin D Testing

The vitamin D test of your blood serum is called 25 (OH) vitamin D. You can get this test at your health-care practitioner's office or by ordering an at-home test kit. Most insurance plans cover all, or most, of the cost of an in-practice vitamin D test.

Once you know your vitamin D3 level, you may want to raise your level to optimal, assuming it is less than 100 ng/mL (250 nmol/L). And please remember that the Vitamin D Wellness Protocol may help you raise and maintain your vitamin D3 level to enjoy improved health.

We have discussed what epigenetic factors and dietary supplementation may affect depression. In the next two chapters we look at depression medications: antidepressants.

Chapter 12

Antidepressant Medications

The natural lifestyle choices discussed in chapter 9 may *reduce the risk* of a major depressive disorder (MDD). However, if your symptoms point to a MDD and/or suicidal thoughts, taking the right antidepressants in accordance with prescription instructions may improve your quality of life, and, in some cases, save your life.

You may recall from chapter 5 how neurotransmitters settle into the brain's synaptic region (think of a lake). These neurotransmitters bind to their transporters/receptors (on the left side of the lake) and travel into the post-synaptic area (the right side of the lake bank).

Antidepressants recycle neurotransmitters by selectively inhibiting their attachment to the transporters. In other words, antidepressants keep an ample supply of neurotransmitters in the synaptic regions (lakes) so we can enjoy the benefits of feeling good.

SSRIs and SNRIs

Two major classes of antidepressants are called SSRI and SNRI. The basic concepts of these medications are not new. For example, the SSRI Prozac has been on the market since the 1960s.

As the name implies, selective serotonin reuptake inhibitors (SSRI) are antidepressants that ensure adequate supplies of serotonin in the brain's synaptic region. Popular SSRIs include citalopram (Celexa), escitalopram (Lexapro), fluoxetine (Prozac), paroxetine (Paxil), and sertraline (Zoloft).

Another popular class of antidepressants is the serotonin–norepinephrine reuptake inhibitors (SNRI). Popular SNRIs include desvenlafaxine (Pristiq), duloxetine (Cymbalta), and venlafaxine (Effexor XR). These medications block the serotonin and norepinephrine receptors so these neurotransmitters stay in the brain's synapse regions (the lakes) to keep us feeling good.

The conventional medical community has debated for years whether SSRIs are more effective than SNRIs. Michael E. Thase, MD, of the University of Pennsylvania's School of Medicine, conducted a review of the controversy between these classes of antidepressants. Citing limitations of randomized controlled trials (RCTs) and meta-analysis, Dr. Thase ascertained that there was no advantage of one class of drugs over the other. His findings were published in a 2008 issue of *Psychopharmacological Bulletin*.

Other Antidepressants

Other classes of antidepressant medication include norepinephrine and dopamine reuptake inhibitors (NDRI), tricyclic antidepressants, and MAO inhibitors (MAOI).

Bupropion (Wellbutrin) is an example of a popular NDRI that is associated with not having the sexual side effects that most antidepressants might cause. Of course, NRDIs tackle both norepinephrine and dopamine by ensuring that these neurotransmitters remain the in "lakes," or the brain's synaptic regions.

An older class of drugs called tricyclic antidepressants may cause more side effects than the newer drugs. These medications are generally not prescribed unless you have initially tried an SSRI without improvement. Examples of tricyclic antidepressants include amitriptyline and doxepin.

Monoamine oxidase inhibitors (MAOIs) carry a lot of baggage for the patient and are not prescribed unless other medication options are exercised. First, MAOIs may have serious side effects. Second, the use of an MAOI requires following a strict diet due to potentially deadly interactions with certain cheeses and fermented foods and some medications including birth control, decongestants, and specific herbal supplements. Finally, MAOIs cannot be combined with other classes of antidepressants.

Future Variations of Antidepressants

Depression is the leading cause of disability in the world. Yet Big Pharma has not provided a major depression-drug breakthrough in almost thirty years!

For what it is worth, Big Pharma is developing a variation of SSRI and SNRI antidepressants that could culminate in taking only one pill a day. The medication under development, referred to as "triple reuptake inhibitors" (TRIs) or serotonin–norepinephrine–dopamine reuptake inhibitors (SNDRIs), focuses on enhancing not only serotonin and norepinephrine synaptic levels but also those for dopamine.

Another possible treatment, inspired by an anesthetic medication called ketamine, is being explored by Big Pharma. Realizing that about 30 percent of depressive persons do not respond well to antidepressants, Big Pharma sees a possible way to treat these people, and treat them quickly so they feel better. (Ketamine is fast-acting, but its duration remains unclear, at least to the public.)

A report published in a July 2017 electronic issue of the *Journal of Medicinal Chemistry* identified SNDRIs as treatment for a "large unmet medical need"—that is, many depression patients also need enhanced dopamine. The author, Dr. Murugaiah A. M. Subbaiah, emphasized that triple uptake inhibitors must be more effective and better tolerated than other antidepressants. He also stated that the therapeutic potential goes beyond depression. Clinical studies include examining the effect of TRIs for patients who have attention deficit hyperactivity disorder (ADHD), binge eating disorder, cocaine addiction, and obesity.

In my opinion, understanding the different types of antidepressants and how they would work with methylation gene variants is paramount to successful treatment. However, when I started seeing a psychiatrist, I asked if he was familiar with genetic mutations and how they may affect depression. His response was nothing short of "hogwash." In other words, conventional medical schools of psychiatry apparently do not focus on the importance of methylation and its genetic variants.

During the initial visit, my psychiatrist recorded the prescription medicines and supplements that I was taking. Then he listened to my description of symptoms and prescribed an antidepressant. For the next twelve months we "tinkered" with different antidepressants until

I felt great on a combination of them. During this "tinkering phase," I was aware of my depression-related gene variants, and found that certain antidepressants worked better than others. At least in my case, antidepressants correlated to depression-related gene variants that apparently were turned on by decades of epigenetic stress.

Serotonin Syndrome

It is worth mentioning again that a rare condition called "serotonin syndrome" could develop if you combine a serotonin (SSRI or SNRI) antidepressant with a monoamine oxidase inhibiting (MAOI) drug. For example, an SSRI increases the amount of serotonin in the brain's synaptic regions (lakes), and a MAOI drug slows the breakdown of serotonin. Hence, serotonin syndrome could arise quickly and cause a wide range of neurological symptoms. Most psychiatrists know to avoid a situation that could culminate in serotonin syndrome. If you are unsure about the combination of prescribed antidepressants, ask your doctor.

In the next chapter I discuss advantages and disadvantages of antidepressant medications.

Chapter 13

Pros and Cons of Antidepressant Medications

Antidepressant medications saved my life—my thoughts and feelings are at peace, and my quality of life has soared to highly functioning. However, it is no secret that antidepressants are associated with side effects and other potentially negative attributes. You need to be aware of both the good and the bad of these prescription medications.

Remember that the biochemistry of antidepressants may fit nicely into the makeup of someone who is seriously depressed and has genetic variants related to depression. I am living proof of the benefits of antidepressants, and believe, if the circumstances are right, that antidepressants can resolve depression symptoms.

Advantages of Antidepressant Medication

They Work! If you are experiencing symptoms of a major depressive disorder (MDD) and have gene mutations associated with depression (see chapter 6), antidepressant drugs may work well. It is paramount for the prescribing physician or psychiatrist to match the correct antidepressant with your symptoms and, ideally, with your methylation-related SNPs.

For the purposes of this chapter, I refer to two major classes of antidepressants: SSRI and SNRI. These medications are designed to ensure an ample supply of depression-related neurotransmitters remain in the brain's synaptic areas to keep us at least reasonably happy.

Cost, Depending on Insurance. If you have health-care insurance that covers the majority of drug costs, the economic impact of buying antidepressants is minimal. For example, I only pay a maximum of ten dollars a month per medication. Considering that SSRIs and SNRIs work well for me, the out-of-pocket costs for the wonderful return are a bargain.

Easy to Take. SSRIs and SNRIs are delivered by easy-to-swallow capsules and tablets that you can take in privacy. No nasty injections or placing drops under the tongue. Without any fanfare or additional medical appointments, you can take your antidepressants with vitamin supplements with your daily breakfast or as directed. Simply easy!

Disadvantages of Antidepressant Medications

They May Not Work! Despite decades of research, antidepressants not only do not work for some folks, they can lead to suicidal ideation or the act itself. Why? First, everyone differs bio-chemically; a treatment that works well for one person might not work well for another. Second, the symptoms may not match the specific antidepressant's mechanisms of action. Third, the antidepressant's properties may not match the gene variants related to the MDD. Finally, the patient might not comply with the instructions for use of the medication.

Side Effects. Antidepressants may lead to a plethora of negative side effects that include headache, weight gain, insomnia, sexual dysfunction, suicidal thoughts, dry mouth, diarrhea, dizziness, nervousness, and agitation. The only negative side effect that I have experienced due to taking several antidepressants at once is weight gain. Given my post-menopausal age and sedentary lifestyle (research and writing go along with sitting at a computer), weight gain is common. And taking antidepressants, as I do, only exacerbates the weight gain.

Cost, Depending on Insurance. If you do not have health-care insurance, or your policy does not cover prescription medications, the monthly cost of the some of the SSRIs and SNRIs could be high.

Potential Lifetime Commitment. When you have an MMD and depression-related gene variants, you most likely would stay on antidepressants for the remainder of your life. If you believe you don't need to stay on antidepressants, you would need to wean yourself off the medication under the prescriber's guidance.

Disadvantage of Drinking Alcohol

Alcohol and antidepressants do not mix. Why? Well, alcohol is a depressant. Drinking it most likely will counteract the benefits of antidepressants, making your symptoms more challenging to treat.

"Yes" or "No" to Antidepressants?

As I am in my sixties, have been diagnosed with depression, and carry some depression-related

SNPs, I do not see myself getting off the anti-depressants that I am taking. For me, antidepressants are effective. They enable me to enjoy an excellent, high-functioning life instead of a miserable life in the abyss of worthlessness and despair. With that said, I am aware that long-terms effects could rear their ugly heads at some point.

While under the care of a psychiatrist, I tried a couple times, under his direction, to stop taking one of the low-dosage antidepressants to no avail. Within a few days, my husband would notice a negative change in my behavior, or I would begin to think depression-like thoughts. Without fail, when going back to the medication, I would feel great. Some psychiatric experts might call my euphoria the "placebo effect."

The study of the placebo effect on psychiatric patients has been examined over the past several decades. As a more recent example, researchers at Columbia University conducted a meta-analysis to examine patients' power of belief in psychiatric treatment. Published in a 2014 issue of the *Journal of Clinical Psychiatry*, the research team concluded that psychiatric treatment changes influence patients' expectations of improvement.

Unfortunately, depression carries social baggage. In the next chapter we look at overcoming the stigma of depression.

Chapter 14

Overcoming the Stigma of Depression

ere we are nearing the third decade of the twenty-first century, and the word "depression" gloomily hangs over society as a label of aberration. Few "normal" people want to deal with the subject of depression, let alone personally experience it.

I think it is ironic that there are so many mental-health-related words or expressions in the English language that, in some cases dating to the nineteenth century, continue to be used in our vernacular. "That's insane...crazy... nuts!" "What is this? An insane asylum?" "He's a total nut job." "She must be mental."

I also find it highly interesting that most people view mental illness in the "shush" category, yet the aforementioned phrases are commonly spoken every day in the United States! But mention that someone actually has depression, and most fall silent, becoming shamed or embarrassed.

Speaking Out About Depression

The stigma of depression spans the globe. However, some people, including well-respected celebrities, are embracing the need to end the silence about depression.

The Duke and Duchess of Cambridge, Prince William and Kate Middleton, and Prince Harry of Wales have proudly founded a mental health charity called "Heads Together." Prior to the 2017 London Marathon, these British royals talked about spearheading a campaign to have "simple conversations" about depression.

Duchess Kate acknowledged that initiating those conversations is often the most difficult part of breaking down the stigma. Her brother-in-law elaborated further by admitting that he "shut down" his emotions for twenty years after the untimely death of his beloved mother, Princess Diana. Prince Harry admitted to *The Telegraph*, "My way of dealing with it was sticking my head in the sand…" He finally sought solace in counseling, and proudly stated, "I've been able to take my work seriously, take my private life seriously, as well, and be able to put blood, sweat and tears into the things that really make a difference."

Furthermore, Oscar-nominated actress Gabourey Sidibe acknowledged that dealing with depression can mean getting outside help. She admitted depression and panic attacks in her 2017 book *This Is Just My Face: Try Not to Stare*. After battling years-long depression,

Sidibe realized that "[depression is] too big for me to just turn around on my own," and she sought a therapist and medical doctor to better manage her mental health.

Award-winning singer and songwriter Demi Lovato told *People* in May 2017, "I'm living well with my mental illness—I am actually functioning like a very happy person would." She also is adamant about fighting the stigma that mood disorders carry, and adds, "I just think mental illness is something people need to learn more about and the stigma needs to be taken away from."

My friend Sheila Hamilton, author of the 2015 book *All the Things We Never Knew: Chasing the Chaos of Mental Illness*, is another crusader for eliminating the stigma of mental illness, including depression. She stated in a May 2016 *Huffington Post* article that she believes, "[B]anishing the stigma around mental illness is the most important civil rights issue of our time. Shame and silence won't improve access to care or improve quality of care. You know what makes a difference? Finding your voice."

Well, I have found my voice by writing *Silent Inheritance* as one of my instruments of communication to the world. Almost everyone inherits at least one genetic variant related to neurotransmitter imbalance, that when turned on by epigenetics, can manifest into depression. There is nothing wrong with that! In fact, this knowledge should empower and inspire people to understand their genetic mutations and learn how to cope with them when necessary.

Chapter 15

Steps Forward to Easing Depression

At this point, you have learned about depression, how genetics and epigenetics can culminate in depression, and how natural solutions and antidepressants can help relieve depression symptoms.

Here are my thoughts on steps to overcome depression:

First, don't beat yourself up. It's not your fault (or your parents', grandparents', and so on) you have depression. Recognize and accept that you may have inherited depression-related gene variants that have been passed down in your family over many generations.

Second, get your DNA tested. Take the easy, at-home Ancestry saliva test to acquire your raw data. Interpret your data by using on-line or medical professional resources. *Silent Inheritance* has provided information on decoding the depression-related gene variants.

Third, based on your methylation gene variants and depression-related symptoms, consider taking a biochemical blood and/or saliva test such as a neurotransmitter test to corroborate your DNA test results and depression symptoms.

Fourth, obtain professional support from your primary-care physician or a psychiatrist. Remember that antidepressant medications are only prescribed by licensed medical professionals.

Fifth, if you prefer to go the natural way, consult a functional doctor or a nurse practitioner who specializes in nutrition and understands how to interpret DNA data.

Sixth, add routine exercise to your life. A 2017 US study concluded that adequate "physical activity diminishes the risk of MDD and suicidal ideation imposed by a genetic [*COMT* rs737865 and rs6265] predisposition."

Seventh, consider enjoying meditation. Ten to fifteen minutes in a quiet place can do wonders for your mind.

Finally, carefully follow the instructions of your professional. If you feel that your treatment is not working properly, immediately contact your mental health professional.

Keep the faith in yourself and your support system including family, friends, medical professionals, and social media help groups. You are not alone. Your path to recovery begins now!

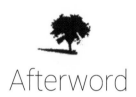

Afterword

Twelve months later...

Sunlight slipped through the office courtyard, highlighting my psychiatrist's delight. Crouched behind a massively intimidating wooden desk, his Irish eyes danced with an apparent infrequent sense of accomplishment: he had treated and healed a patient—me!

Before the psychiatrist escorted me to the patient checkout area, he rose from his seat and wholeheartedly shook my hand. The smiling doctor proudly announced to his reception staff, "No further appointments!"

The terrible weight of depression was gone. Although I remain on a few antidepressants (subsequently prescribed by my primary-care physician), I am living a peaceful and content, high-functioning life. And now, I sing my song of *Silent Inheritance,* with great hope that my words will inspire you or a loved one to find relief from depression.

Appendix A

Methylation Cycles

My thoughts about methylation are tucked into this appendix. Some readers may find this too technical, so it is here for reference.

Methionine Cycle

The **methionine cycle** processes homocysteine to generate methionine, a vital amino acid, into SAMe (S-adenosyl methionine), a chemical produced in the liver that can be an effective and well-tolerated treatment for depression. The adequate intake of B vitamins from diet or supplements is required to trigger

ATP (adenosine triphosphate) concentrations in our cells to activate the methionine.

Homocysteine levels must be carefully balanced by adequate quantities of specific B vitamins. Approximately one-half of homocysteine is recycled back into methionine (remethylation), and the other half is converted via transsulfuration into a beneficial amino acid called cysteine.

The bifurcated recycling process depends on availability of specific B vitamins. Remethylation cannot occur without folate (vitamin B9) and vitamin B12, and transsulfuration cannot happen without vitamin B6. If these B vitamins are deficient, dangerous levels of homocysteine can accumulate in the body and damage the lining of the arteries, potentially increasing the risk of heart disease.

Folate Cycle

The **folate cycle** processes a water-soluble vitamin called folate (B9) as well as B2 (riboflavin), B6, and B12 to synthesize DNA and metabolize amino acids, or protein building blocks. Green leafy vegetables are the primary dietary source for folate. This is a good time to note that the *folate cycle needs folate*, not the synthetic folic acid commonly found in processed food.

The *MTHFR* genes are involved in the folate cycle. During this cycle, the reduced form of folate called 5-MTHF joins vitamin B12 and another molecule (methionine synthase) to convert homocysteine back to methionine. As we know, this conversion process is key to maintaining a healthy cardiovascular system, i.e., excess homocysteine can increase the risk of coronary artery disease.

BH4 Cycle

The **BH4 cycle** is the process that focuses on the balance of dopamine and serotonin neurotransmitters. BH4, or tetrahydrobiopterin, helps convert tryptophan to serotonin and tyrosine to dopamine. In addition, adequate levels of BH4 are vital to the urea cycle.

GEEK SPEAK: Adequate BH4 is essential to rid our bodies of ammonia. Two molecules of BH4 are required to clean one molecule of ammonia in order to be eliminated by our liver and kidneys.

But only one molecule of BH4 versus one molecule of ammonia yields peroxynitrate, a substance that can damage DNA.

Unfortunately, zero molecules of BH4 versus one molecule of ammonia produce superoxide, which can act as a free radical when connected to an unpaired electron.

Urea Cycle

Finally, the **urea cycle** acts as our waste-processing plant. Enzymes in the urea cycle process toxic chemicals, including ammonia, in order for them to be eliminated from our bodies. Adequate BH4 is essential to the smooth operation of the urea cycle and is integral for producing nitric oxide to maintain cardiovascular health.

Appendix B

Other Depressive-Related Disorders

Could we be predisposed to other mental health disorders, specifically anxiety, bipolar disorder, and obsessive-compulsive disorder? The answer is "yes."

These mental health disorders are indeed connected to depression. With the exception of the SNPs related to anxiety, you can recognize gene variants that are common to depression mutations.

Anxiety

Depression and anxiety are often thought of interchangeably because they share similar symptoms and are often treated in the same manner. A person with an anxiety disorder may suffer fear, panic, and, yes, anxiety in situations where most people would not feel threatened or anxious.

A couple of gene variants related to anxiety come to mind: *RGS2* (rs4606) and *TPH2* (rs4570625).

Bipolar Disorder

Bipolar disorder is the extreme opposite of depression. Bipolar behavior entails symptoms of mania. In other words, a bipolar person may exhibit excessive euphoria, grandiose elation, and impulsive behaviors such as going on shopping sprees or engaging in promiscuous sex.

Bipolar-related gene variants include *DAO* (rs2070586 and rs3741775) as well as *COMT*

H62H and *COMT V158M* gene mutations (rs4633 and rs4680, respectively).

OCD

Obsessive-compulsive disorder (OCD) is closely linked to anxiety. For the first time, however, in 2013, the American Psychiatric Association treated OCD separately from anxiety in the *DSM-V*.

Behavior of individuals exhibiting OCD includes hoarding and self-mutilation such as skin picking.

The *MAO-A R297R* (rs6323) "warrior" gene mutation is commonly associated with OCD behavior. As I mentioned earlier, a variant in this gene involves an imbalance of serotonin, dopamine, and norepinephrine.

Appendix C

The Importance of
Homocysteine

Naturally produced in your body, a chemical substance called homocysteine often becomes elevated due to age, diet, and genetic disposition. If your homocysteine is high, you are at an increased risk of developing depression.

Homocysteine is an amino acid (a building block of protein) naturally produced in the body from methionine. Healthy amounts of homocysteine are vital in protein metabolism. However, homocysteine levels must be carefully balanced by adequate quantities of folate, vitamin B6, and vitamin B12.

During healthy methylation, about half of the homocysteine is recycled back into methionine (remethylation), and the other half is converted into a beneficial amino acid called cysteine (transsulfuration). This bifurcated process is dependent on specific B vitamins.

Remethylation cannot occur without folate and vitamin B12. Transsulfuration cannot happen without vitamin B6. If these B vitamins are deficient, dangerous levels of homocysteine can accumulate in the body and cause a variety of maladies including depression.

What is a Healthy Homocysteine Level?

Homocysteine levels are easily evaluated by a simple test of blood plasma. Health-care practitioners can order a homocysteine test. But guess what? We are not routinely tested for homocysteine. In fact, I never had been tested for this important amino acid until I requested the test from my primary-care physician.

To further exacerbate the issue of homocysteine evaluation, many clinical testing laboratories consider a healthy homocysteine value between 5 and up to 15 μmol/L. However, the upper limit of this range is highly misleading. A score of 6 μmol/L or less is optimal for homocysteine. High levels of homocysteine may indicate an increased risk for depression. Not all depressed persons have elevated homocysteine scores, and not all people with high homocysteine are depressed.

Appendix D

Menopause and Depression

My depression only set in after I was through menopause. Having connected the dots, I believe that my estrogen levels were affected by gene variants involved in this hormone's metabolism. After decades of stress similar to what was described in chapter 9, my gene mutations associated with estrogen metabolism were apparently turned on.

In my case, I am heterozygous for the *CYP1A2*, *CYP1B1*, and *CYP19A1* gene variants that are directly involved in the processing of two forms of estrogen: estrone (E1) and estradiol (E2).

Due to the expression of these *CYP* gene variants, my body was producing less estrogen than someone without these mutations. Less estrogen is correlated with less serotonin. Thus, I lacked adequate amounts of serotonin, probably contributing to depression symptoms.

I also note that *COMT* gene variants rs4680 and rs4633 may affect the processing of E1. (For the record, I am negative for tested *COMT* gene variants.) In other words, your female hormones may be affected by having both *COMT* and *CYP* gene mutations.

If you are in perimenopause, menopause, or are postmenopausal AND experiencing the symptoms discussed in chapter 2, I suggest getting your hormones checked by saliva or blood testing (see chapter 7) as well as genetic testing. By analyzing your symptoms, biochemistry, and genetics, your medical professional can advise you how to bioidentically balance your female hormones vis-à-vis your genetic profile.

Appendix E

The Near Future of Genetics

The near future of genetics—gene editing and repair—is here, but its approach continues to be carefully considered. Of course, the possibility of modifying genes conjures up a plethora of questions surrounding moral issues. Nonetheless, the scientific research has culminated in the reality of gene-editing technology.

Over the past few years, a genetic-editing technique called CRISPR (Clustered Regularly Interspaced Short Palindromic Repeats) has taken the mainstream news by storm. Scientists can now target a specific DNA sequence and readily make repairs. Please note that, at the time of this writing, CRISPR research has been limited to the laboratory.

A study published in the July 2015 issue of the scientific journal *Protein & Cell* rocked the science world. The lead author, Oxford University professor Julian Savulescu, and his team stated,

> Gene editing technologies have enormous potential as a therapeutic tool in the fight against disease...Gene editing could significantly lower [this] disease burden thereby benefitting billions of people around the world over time. To intentionally refrain from engaging in life-saving research is to be morally responsible for the foreseeable, avoidable deaths of those who could have benefitted. Research into gene-editing is not an option, it is a moral necessity.

Editing and repairing specific genetic *mutations* hopefully will soon become a reality for depressive patients. Think of what gene editing could do to resolve a major depression disorder. For example, editing and repair of the *MAO-A R297R* gene variant could result in a balance of neurotransmitters, transforming the "warrior" gene to one of potential contentment!

Bibliography

Aseervatham, GS et al. "Environmental factors and unhealthy lifestyle influence oxidative stress in humans—an overview." *Environ Sci Pollut Res Int.* 2013 Jul;20(7):4356-69.

Braly, James and Holford, Patrick. *The H Factor Solution*. Basic Health Publications, Inc. 2008.

Brogan, Kelly. *A Mind of Your Own*. Harper Wave. 2016.

Burns, David D. *Feeling Good: The New Mood Therapy*. Harper. 1999.

Chirinos, DA et al. "Depressive symptom profiles, cardio-metabolic risk and inflammation: Results from the MIDUS study." *Psychoneuroendochrinology.* 2017 Apr 29;82:17-25.

Doudna, Jennifer and Sternberg, Samuel. *A Crack in Creation*. Houghton Miffin Harcourt. 2017.

Evrensel A and Ceylan ME. "The Gut-Brain Axis: The Missing Link in Depression." *Clin Psychopharmacol Neurosci*. 2015 Dec 31;13(3):239-44.

Frankel, Paul. *The Methylation Miracle*. St. Martin's. 1999.

Gibbons, A., "Tracking the Evolutionary History of the "Warrior" Gene." *Science*. 2004 May 7;304(5672):818.

Gougeon, L et al. "Intakes of folate, vitamin B6 and B12 and risk of depression in community-dwelling older adults: the Quebec Longitudinal Study on Nutrition and Aging." *Eur J Clin Nutr*. 2016 Mar; 70(3):380-5.

Gougen, L et al. "A prospective evaluation of the depression-nutrient intake reverse causality hypothesis in a cohort of community-dwelling older Canadians." *Br J Nutr.* 2017 Apr;117(7):1032-1041.

Greenblatt James M. *Breakthrough Depression Solution*. Sunrise River Press. 2016.

Greenblatt, James M and Brogan, Kelly. *Integrative Therapies for Depression*. CRC Press. 2016.

Hyde, CL et al. "Identification of 15 genetic loci associated with risk of major depression in individuals of European decent." *Nature Genetics*. 2016 Sep;48(9):1031-6.

Hyman, Mark. *The UltraMind Solution*. Scribner. 2009.

Jiang, W et al. "Association between *MTHFR C677T* polymorphism and depression: a meta-analysis in the Chinese population." *Psychol Health* Med. 2016 Sep;21(6):675-85.

Jimenez, KM et al. "*Val158Met* polymorphism in the *COMT* gene is associated with hypersomnia and mental health-related quality of life in Columbian sample." *Neurosci Lett.* 2017 Feb 22;644:43-47.

Kharrazian, Datis. *Why Isn't My Brain Working?* Elephant Press. 2013.

Knueppel, A et al. "Sugar intake from sweet food and beverages, common mental disorder and depression: prospective findings from the Whitehall II study." *Sci Rep.* 2017 Jul 27;7(1):6287.

Pacholok, Sally and Stuart, Jeffrey. *Could It Be B12?* Quill Driver Books. 2011.

Polak, MA. et al. "Serum 25-hydroxyvitamin D concentrations and depressive symptoms among young adult men and women." *Nutrients.* 2014 Oct 28;6(11):4720-30.

Rozycka, A. et al. "The *MAO, COMT, MTHFR,* and *ESR1* gene polymorphisms are associated with the risk of depression in menopausal women." *Maturitas.* 2016 Feb;84:42-54.

Rutherford, BR. et al. "The role of patient expectancy in placebo and nocebo effects in antidepressant trials." *J Clin Psychiatry.* 2014 Oct;75(10):1040-6.

Savulescu, J et al. "The moral imperative to continue gene editing research on human embryos." *Protein Cell.* 2015 Jul;6(7):476-479.

Slopien, R. et al. "The *c.1460C>T* polymorphism of *MAO-A* is associated with the risk of depression in postmenopausal women." *ScientificWorldJournal.* 2012;2012:194845.

Subbaiah, MAM, "Triple Uptake Inhibitors as Potential Therapeutics for Depression and Other Disorders: Design Paradigm and Developmental Challenges." *J Med Chem*, 2017 Jul 21. Epub.

Taylor, MK et al. "A genetic factor for major depression and suicidal ideation is mitigated by physical activity." *Psychiatry Res.* 2017 Mar;249:304-306.

Thase, ME. "Are SNRIs more effective than SSRIs? A review of the current state of the controversy." *Psychopharmacol Bull.* 2008;31(2):58-85.

Walsh, William J. *Nutrient Power.* Skyhorse Publishing. 2012, 2014.

Wu, YL et al. "Association between *MTHFR C677T* polymorphism and depression: An updated meta-analysis of 26 studies." *Prog Neuropsychopharmocol Biol Psychiatry.* 2013 Oct 1;46:78-85.

Yasko, Amy. *Feel Good: Nutrigenomics.* NRI, LLC. 2014.

Index

Acknowledgments

The support of my family, including that of my wonderful husband, Dave, helped me get through those long days of researching the scientific literature and writing this book.

I would like to thank my primary-care physician and my psychiatrist for helping me achieve a state of contentment and even happiness. Without your support, I know *Silent Inheritance* would not have come to fruition.

Special thanks to Cheryl Strayed, *New York Times* number-one best-selling author of *Wild*. In 2015, I was fortunate to study writing under

Cheryl's sage tutelage. Her self-confidence and courage inspired me to tell my story about what had been the unthinkable for me: depression.

The cover of *Silent Inheritance* is a product of a superb graphic design professional named Shannon Bodie of BookWise Design in Oregon. The visual magic performed by Shannon and her team enhances the feel of this book.

I would also like to thank the women and men who have devoted themselves to seeking viable solutions to depression. Millions of us need the fruition of your research.

Finally, I would like to express gratitude to people who are brave enough to help overcome the stigma of depression by publicly acknowledging their depression. Thank you.

About the Author

Susan "Sue" Rex Ryan was born and raised in the Philadelphia, Pennsylvania area. She earned a bachelor of science degree at Georgetown University, concentrating on languages and linguistics. Sue also holds a master of science degree from the US military's National War College in Washington, DC. In addition, she has earned scores of Continuing Medical Education (CME) credits from accredited US medical programs approved by, inter alia, The American Academy of Family Physicians.

Her debut book, entitled *Defend Your Life*, discusses the many health benefits of vitamin D and has garnered global accolades as an Amazon bestseller. In addition, *Defend Your Life* won a prestigious Mom's Choice Award, an international awards program that recognizes authors and others for their efforts in creating quality family-friendly media products.

In 2015, Sue founded a private vitamin D support group on social media that has nearly 15,000 members and established her Vitamin D Protocol. By communicating with members from around the world, she learned that many endure methylation issues that adversely affect their brain health. By connecting the dots with extensive medical literature research combined with her own experiences, Sue wrote this, her second book, entitled *Silent Inheritance*.

By writing *Silent Inheritance*, Sue's sincere wish is that everyone—women and men of all ages—improve their mental quality of life by balancing specific brain chemicals. Since balancing her neurotransmitters and following her Vitamin D Wellness Protocol, Sue's mental quality of life has significantly improved. She hopes that your life as well the lives of your loved ones and friends will benefit from the information contained in *Silent Inheritance*.

Sue and her husband, Dave, reside in the sunny suburbs of beautiful Las Vegas, Nevada. They enjoy traveling to visit family and friends, as well as experiencing life in far-flung locations including Sri Lanka, Easter Island, and French Polynesia.

Follow Sue's commentary on Twitter @VitD3Sue. She welcomes your visit to her website smilinsuepubs.com, which is replete with her blog articles about health topics.

Made in the
USA
Monee, IL